To Sue,

I hope you find this little book useful.

love,
Nadia

August 2017

HOW DID I GET THESE?

NADIA SMITH

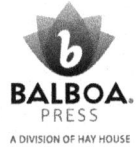

BALBOA PRESS
A DIVISION OF HAY HOUSE

Copyright © 2017 Nadia Smith.

All rights reserved. No part of this book may be used or reproduced by any means, graphic, electronic, or mechanical, including photocopying, recording, taping or by any information storage retrieval system without the written permission of the author except in the case of brief quotations embodied in critical articles and reviews.

Balboa Press books may be ordered through booksellers or by contacting:

Balboa Press
A Division of Hay House
1663 Liberty Drive
Bloomington, IN 47403
www.balboapress.com
1 (877) 407-4847

Because of the dynamic nature of the Internet, any web addresses or links contained in this book may have changed since publication and may no longer be valid. The views expressed in this work are solely those of the author and do not necessarily reflect the views of the publisher, and the publisher hereby disclaims any responsibility for them.

The author of this book does not dispense medical advice or prescribe the use of any technique as a form of treatment for physical, emotional, or medical problems without the advice of a physician, either directly or indirectly. The intent of the author is only to offer information of a general nature to help you in your quest for emotional and spiritual well-being. In the event you use any of the information in this book for yourself, which is your constitutional right, the author and the publisher assume no responsibility for your actions.

Any people depicted in stock imagery provided by Thinkstock are models, and such images are being used for illustrative purposes only. Certain stock imagery © Thinkstock.

Print information available on the last page.

ISBN: 978-1-5043-8369-1 (sc)
ISBN: 978-1-5043-8370-7 (e)

Library of Congress Control Number: 2017910818

Balboa Press rev. date: 08/10/2017

Dedication

To my formidable mother, Diane Marcus de Nekludoff, known to me as Mamy, to my cousins as Tante Didi, and in the latter part of her years either as "Mrs N" or "Grand-Mere".

ACKNOWLEDGEMENT

A great big "Thank You" to our sons, Ashley and Laurie, for helping us open our eyes to Spirituality, and for helping us raise our awareness that merging our material and physical selves with our energetic and spiritual beings really elevates our lives on earth to an infinite source of successful supply on demand.

I am so grateful to all my students and clients, past and present, for having had so much trust in me and encouraging me to continue my search in developing our Human Inheritance of self-healing, True to our Roots Qi Gong, and for having been my "Guinea-Pigs"!

To my husband, Roger Smith, for not totally losing his rag with my inept computer skills, and for being forever supportive of all my enthusiastic projects throughout our married life. Especially I thank him for being my Personal Assistant with regards to the production of this book, as without his professional skills as a computer buff, I would have been lost.

And last but not least, to my own body for the amount of "abuse" it suffered before I saw the light, which I am now able to share with you.

FOREWORD

By Josephine Cropper

When I think of Nadia, I always smile. She is a little powerhouse of a woman; a bundle of joy with a zest for life.

I met Nadia some years ago when we were on a training course together. She was one of those people who immediately intrigued me. I felt as though she had many secrets to reveal, and I wanted to know more! Nadia has had an unusual life, having a Belgian mother and Indian father. In this book you will not only read about the body, and how events have impacted on her body and how to overcome those issues for yourself, but there is also a fascinating life story.

> What happens to a little child when they are abused by their parents? They cannot run away, as is the natural human reaction if a predator threatens you! They cannot fight as their parents are bigger and it is disrespectful, as I was taught! The next instinctive reaction is to "freeze"! "Forever standing to attention", as we never know when the hand may strike again, or the words will hurt your soul! Subconsciously setting this "iron corset" up, as the core muscles, the psoas or the "Messenger of the Soul" (as described by Liz Koch), shorten, get tighter or better still "freeze".

Nadia Smith

Today we accept that there is a powerful mind-body connection through which emotional, mental, social, spiritual and behavioural factors can directly affect our health. In this book Nadia shows us how, by following Louise Hay's example from "Heal your Body", our mind, health and body are connected. She describes the impact on her own life and then gives us real-life examples of what this can mean for our bodies and overall wellbeing.

> "Six-pack Nad" had to learn the "art of softening" to help her body heal and needed to understand that it was all right to show vulnerability.

> The hardness approach had broken my body, and now I needed to learn how to help it better. I felt I had nothing to move forward to, which relates totally with what Louise Hay describes.

Nadia looks at life from a practical point of view, asking what she can do to help herself in a situation and how she can keep positive and look after herself and her body no matter how difficult the situation may be. She had to cope with the diagnosis of cerebral palsy for their first child, and the death of their second child.

> That day and night I spent either wandering around helplessly in the cattle-shed type ward, with wind howling through, wafting smells of cabbage all around us, and visiting my little boy in his starched hospital gown inside the incubator, with cockroaches running around inside it.

> In the meantime, we continued to gain experiences on survival, as within the first year of our life in the Eastern Province of Zambia,

> the water stopped flowing. My new vegetable garden dried out and we programmed ourselves to wake up at 3AM.

Nadia is truly dedicated to helping people have better lives, and is an expert in Qi Gong, having devised her own version called "True to our Roots Qi Gong". Qi Gong comes from the Chinese words for "Energy" and "Work". She is a Tui Na master practitioner and qualified Qi Gong instructor with over 25 years' experience. She has studied with various Qi Gong masters and has trained at the Xi Yuan University Hospital in Beijing.

She has been practising traditional Chinese healing arts in her clinic since 1999, and her skills include Cranio-Sacral Therapy, Skeletal Realignment, Psoas Muscle Release and Trauma Release Exercises. She has special expertise in hip replacement maintenance.

However, there is so much more to this book; it will take you on a heart-warming, interesting and uplifting journey.

> In July 2009,… I did another Core Awareness course with Liz Koch. This was most valuable as she introduced us to Esther Gokhale's book, "Eight Steps to a Painfree Back". This book changed my life and eased pain that no therapist had been able to help me with.
>
> The miracle of this was how I addressed my posture, especially when standing and walking.

As a psychotherapist I often hear the details of people's lives. Nadia, however, has a particularly rich and heart-warming story to tell. Despite her turbulent past, where many would have given up, she lives life with humour, kindness and ingenuity.

> Very often we went weeks without electricity, we learned how to use the local charcoal fires, which were cylindrical shaped and the size of a large paint pot. Once I cooked food for 36 people on two of those! Whenever we had a power cut for more than three days, we would cook the entire contents of the freezer and have a party for our local friends! It was a great excuse to socialize!
>
> It was at that time that despite still being a Fitness instructor, since 1990 I had also started practising Qi Gong – Chinese Healing movements, which is a totally different approach to Western health and fitness. It is an art which accesses and cultivates internal energy rather than expending it. So, it was this gentle practice which assisted in my gradual softening and trusting more in the natural state of being, one which as a growing child I had always observed from my African peers, who were always cheerful and happy, despite having very little material wealth.

She has the ability to paint the picture so you are there alongside her, even in the most bizarre situations. You can almost feel her breath.

Nadia is one of those rare people we meet in life who truly does inspire. She allows her vulnerability to show, and she uses it to inform her clients' lives, and to help their bodies unlock from the past.

> Look into your past and retrace the years to find what happened to you primarily, to have given you, for example low self-esteem or self-worth. Who were the first people in your life who may have criticised you, or didn't show you the love any small child needs and deserves?

How Did I Get These?

> *Then begin to undo these negative issues by learning to look at yourself in the mirror with love rather than dislike or hatred. Louise Hay's book "You Can Heal Your Life" will give you a wonderful insight on how to begin to heal your own life.*
>
> *When I was a fitness instructor teaching gruelling high and hard impact aerobics, (I was regarded as such a tough teacher that a big guy who was captain of a local rugby team, asked me to give them physical training sessions!), I also started to incorporate the gentle Qi Gong forms into my daily practice and a state of confusion started to arise within my psyche! What was best for me? Western keep fit which gave me a high, or Eastern Qi Gong which made me calm?*
>
> *Allowing the body to move instinctively, however, gives it the opportunity to soften, release the tension, help the blood to flow where it was stuck and heal itself.*

When you've read the book, you will want to re-read it.

I feel sure there are many more events to tell us. Nadia, we await your second book!

Josephine Cropper is one of a mere handful of psychotherapists in the UK to have been awarded a TRE® qualification. This is the ground-breaking treatment for stress, anxiety and post-traumatic stress disorder.

She is based in Horwich, Bolton, Lancashire and has been treating clients for more than 15 years as *JMC Psychotherapy*, and her TRE® qualification is the latest in a line of accolades which include being named as one of 2014's 'Inspirational Women in Bolton' by the *Women in*

Nadia Smith

Neighbourhoods group and receiving a nomination for an Enterprise Vision Award in 2013. She is also a member of the UK Council of Psychotherapy and published author of the book *From Trauma to Freedom*.

She holds a Master of Science degree in psychotherapy from the University of Wales Medical College and has qualifications in Transactional Analysis, pastoral and clinical counselling, EFT (Emotional Freedom Technique), Trauma Therapy and Body Therapy.

Before establishing her own practice, she spent 15 years in management in the textile industry. She gained a Business Studies Degree and was responsible for a budget of £25 million.

Drawing on years of experience in organisations such as the NHS, a women's refuge, a mental health charity and mediation services, she now focuses on her psychotherapy practice.

As a keen pianist she is acutely aware of how stress in the body affects potential for any musician, and is a leading expert in this field.

www.jmcpsychotherapy.com

PREFACE

"How Did I Get These?" is about my agonizing search as to why I developed osteo-arthritis in both my hips, and ending up with two metal hip replacements.

As a result of many lightbulb moments and studying with inspiring teachers, I begun to understand that my body was crying out for my love and attention.

I hope by sharing some of my own life's adventures it will help you to understand your own health story better, and hopefully you too can become your own detective in order to figure out why you may have health issues as a result of emotional challenges.

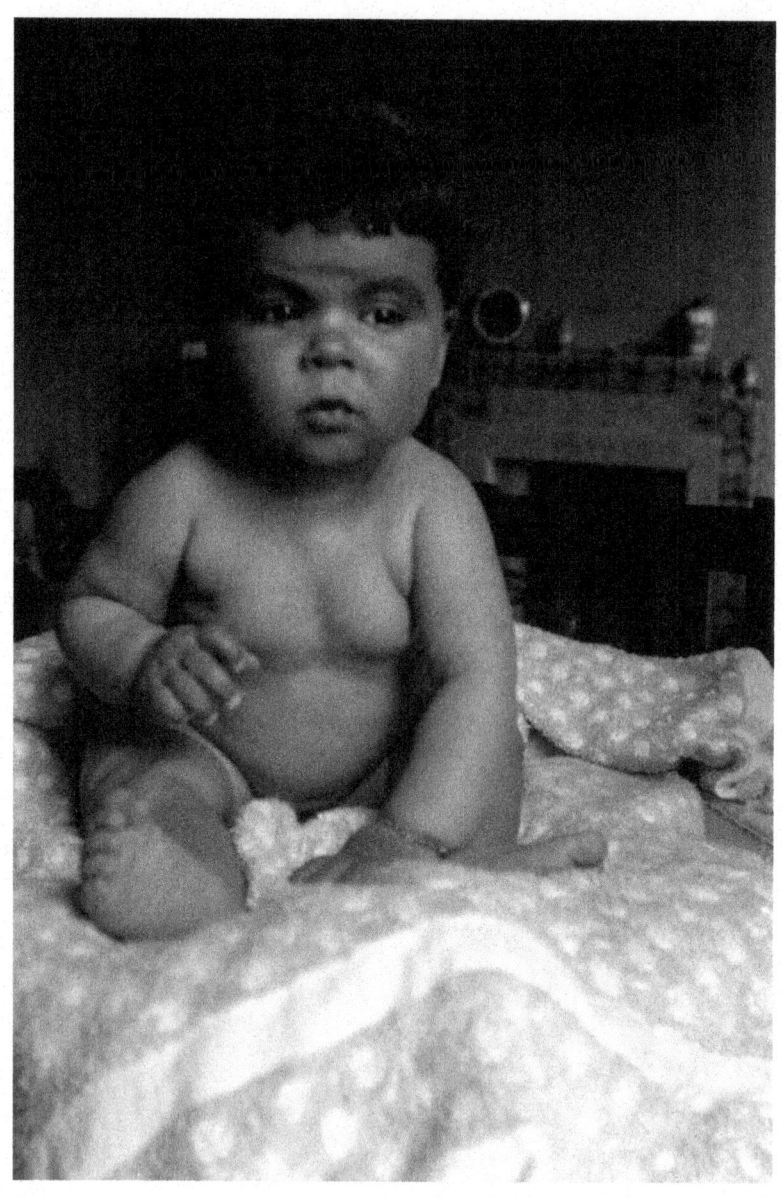

Nadia in England, 1953

INTRODUCTION

Arthritis:

    "Feeling unloved – criticism, resentment"

    ("Heal your Body", Louise Hay)

It all began in the year of 1952, when a little half Asian/European baby girl was born to a young Belgian woman and a young man from the Punjab.

"I hired a detective to photograph your father and me in bed together, so I had proof to divorce my first husband!", a revelation my mother made to me when I was 52 years of age!

My parents had a registry office marriage just one week before my birth. So, I was a means to an end and thus began my life under the iron rule of my very controlling mother.

My dear reader, you may have picked up this little handbook because you need the answers to how to maintain your new hip sockets? The only way I can share this knowledge with you is by making my story of discovery a bit more personal. This was by no means an easy task! Perhaps you will find a correlation with your own life story.

In 1990, at the height of my Fitness Instructor career, when I was 38 years of age, my lovely and wise GP told me: "My dear, your left hip has the onset of osteo-arthritis!" "This could not be right!", my ego argued, "I'm far too young, this only happens to old people!"

So, I left her surgery in total disbelief, and this is where my journey of Self-Denial began.

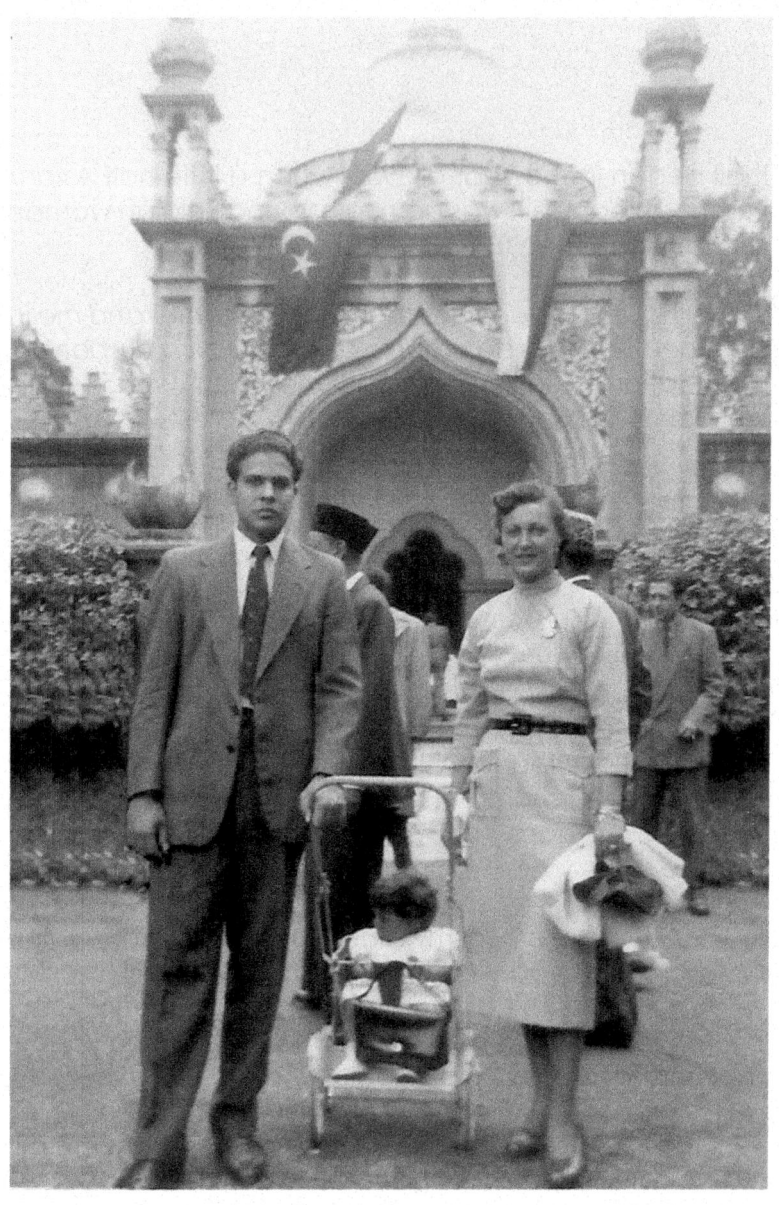

My parents and I in front of Woking mosque after their Muslim wedding, 1953

LESSON 1
SELF-DENIAL

Self-denial

From 1990 to 2005 began my inner battle. I searched for external miracle cures to "fix" my gradually worsening lower back pain, the "referred" pain shooting down my left inner thigh to the knee and eventually affecting the left ankle too.

As a Fitness Instructor I was very fit and even got nicknamed "Six-pack Nad"! That made me very proud, as the stronger I became physically, the less I could get hurt... or so I thought!

The pain came and went thanks to the multitude of therapists I saw and received treatments from: chiropractors, Qi Gong Masters/Doctors, Osteopaths, Physiotherapists, Tui Na practitioners, Acupuncturists, and Massage therapists. I even had my back "cello-taped" for a long-haul flight. The list is endless and everyone helped, but the searing pain always returned.

In 1997 after occasionally appearing at my aerobic classes with a walking stick, I decided to retire and diversify my career to follow the course of Traditional Chinese Medical healing arts.

Everything changed with my first Alexander Technique lesson in 2003, when my teacher told me to halt all physical exercise. This was equivalent to telling a heroin addict to stop the drug instantly without substitute! I suffered from "cold turkey" and my ego was shot to pieces. What kept me "looking and feeling good" all needed to stop! I had to allow the contracted muscles to soften and find their natural place again, as my Alexander Technique teacher advised me.

By 1999 I had become a practitioner in the Chinese Healing Arts myself, and if anyone with menopausal symptoms would come for advice, one of the things I would have recommended would have been exercise of

LESSON 1

some type. Yet, here I was, having to stop all my habitual activities while going through the menopause myself!

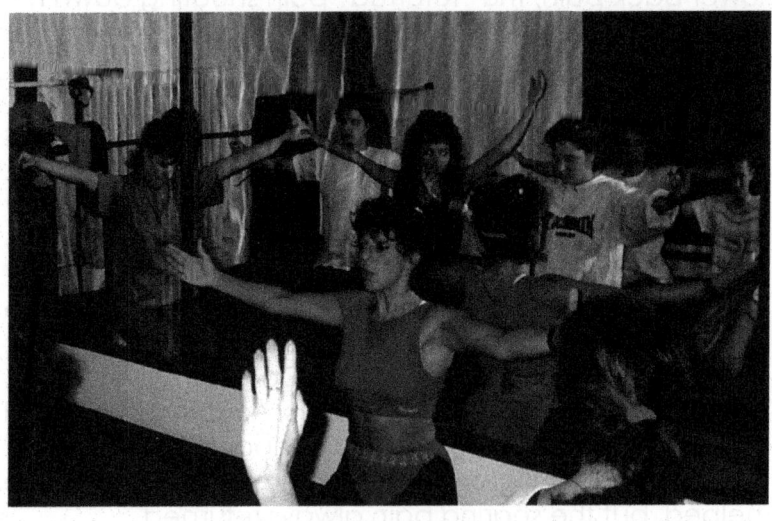

Teaching Aerobics in Budapest, 1992

My physique altered gradually, and I started to put on weight, my left leg started to lose tone and my right leg was always leading when walking. By 2001 I walked with a constant limp.

In 2004 thanks to my Alexander Technique teacher we both attended "The Psoas Muscle Intensive" course, which was a 12 hours exploration of the iliopsoas muscle complex with Liz Koch (www.coreawareness.com).

Those two days opened "lock gates" for me, like a huge lightbulb moment, which to this day continues to flow with the new discoveries about mankind through myself.

During this workshop I had a major emotional jolt through some of the gentle exploratory physical work we did – I was reminded of a four and half years long physically and emotionally abusive relationship I had with a young man I thought was the love of my life. During that relationship, I endured drunken beatings, attempts at strangulations, physical and emotional threats, rape at knife point in Italy by two locals, while the boyfriend cowered from them, his aborted baby, all while he two-timed me with various other girls. He threatened me so much that I lived in constant fear of him, but too afraid to leave him or involve other people out of shame! This really made me understand why women are afraid to leave abusive relationships.

The universe offered a gap for us, when he travelled to Australia to visit his relatives, which helped me to try and rebuild my life in Belgium for a while.

Although I finally ended that relationship to go out with my husband and soul-mate, I never questioned the abuse I suffered until this workshop. A surge of anger and tears arose in me at the injustice of behaviour from this ex-boyfriend, and "How dare he have treated me this way?" As this realisation awoke in me it was accompanied by a deep but all over bodily trembling. How could I have allowed this to happen to me!!

The psoas muscle, connected to our fight/flight/freeze reflex, woke up in me and started to release, which is what we were learning during this two-day workshop.

What a revelation! My body had held this deep-seated, unexpressed fear since 1971 . . . or perhaps gradually since 1952?

An awakening occurred deep within me, which showed me that the osteo-arthritis I had been diagnosed with may not just have been through a physical symptom. This could well be through deeply held fear, which caused the muscles to freeze and become rigid.

LESSON 1

It dawned on me that I was hiding behind my Fitness Instructor's iron harness in order to keep control of my emotions - "not to get hurt". Keeping fit had become my "nu-nu"! All at the cost of my health.

During my career change I also heard and read a lot of alternative "new age" explanations and reasons why we act/react the way we do, in order to cope with life. One was that we attract situations and people to ourselves which or who repeat familiar patterns with which we are accustomed to.

My big question was "How come I attracted such an abusive man into my young life, as a 19-year old? Where did this abusive familiarity come from?"

Again, this realization occurred as a "light bulb" moment, still under the title of "self-denial"... MY MOTHER!! Not till I was 51 years old did I suddenly understand that I had been living under my mother's "iron rod"! Until then I had always been afraid of her – I hankered after her approval, I pussy-footed around her whenever we were together in order to please her, and I totally put her on a pedestal. I believed everything she told me, despite the fact that both ex-boyfriend and my husband disproved her. I protected and defended her fiercely, and yet she never had a kind word to say to me! Nothing was ever good enough for my mother.

1958.

My mother left my father when I was six years old and she took me with her. We lived in Belgian Congo, in the bush at that time. We returned to Bruges, Belgium (mum's home town), and when I was eight, my father visited for the last time. Then they divorced and I never saw him again until I was in my mid-thirties.

Self-denial

It seemed from the divorce time that I remember – or better my body remembers – that my mother stopped loving me. Despite my forever cheerful disposition, she'd always find a reason to either punish me, hit me hard on the back of my head or laugh at me when I cried!

What happens to a little child when they are abused by their parents? They cannot run away, as is the natural human reaction if a predator threatens you! They cannot fight as their parents are bigger and it is disrespectful, as I was taught! The next instinctive reaction is to "freeze"! "Forever standing to attention", as we never know when the hand may strike again, or the words will hurt your soul! Subconsciously setting this "iron corset" up, as the core muscles, the psoas or the "Messenger of the Soul" (as described by Liz Koch), shorten, get tighter or better still "freeze".

"Oh, my goodness… my mother is my abuser!" What an awful, but astonishing realization was that!

I suddenly understood why my lower back had become so rigid, to the point of deformity, and was diagnosed with lordosis or "sway back"

1965. Belgium before leaving for Kenya.

My mother showed me this contraption, like a small nappy with an elasticated belt and told me in an embarrassed way that I'd be needing this soon, as every month little teenage girls bled for a few days, and that this event needed to be recorded monthly, and three days taken off for the next month so that I could be preparing myself to wear this nappy-like contraption. It was best that I didn't tell anyone and then got punished for sharing this mortifying secret with my younger cousin!

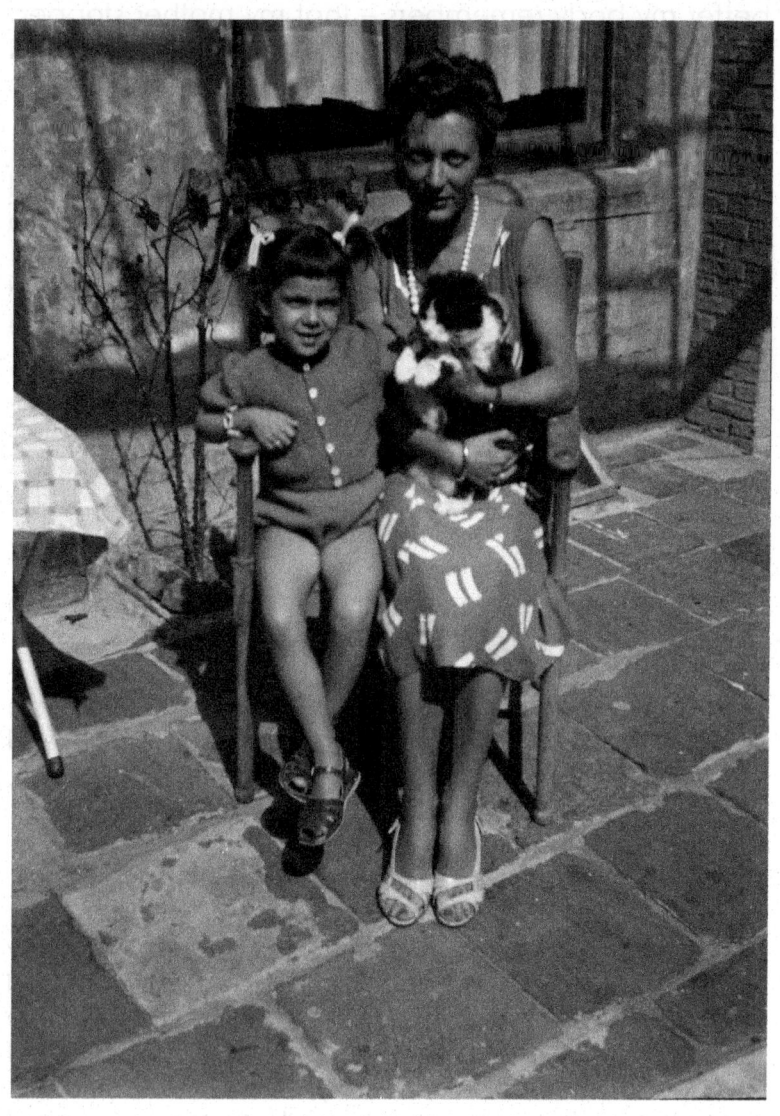

Mum, me and the cat, in Bruges 1956

Self-denial

My mother timed it right as the first occurrence happened during a sewing class at school in Bruges, a week later!

Suddenly growing up into a teenager became something to be really ashamed of, especially as it seemed I had to learn to walk with a nappy between my legs at the cost of people noticing my strange gait! One advantage was not having to shower after our weekly one hour's Physical Education class!

Menstruation coincided with the appearance of "unnecessary" hair in my armpits and "other" places – in utter shame and disgust at myself I used to secretly use my mother's hand hair clippers to remove these few little hairs. These clippers used to tear the hair out from this sensitive area and was quite painful, so I was greatly relieved when meeting my savvy new girlfriends in Kenya that same year, who introduced me to the wonders of the razorblade!

Until our son's birth, my monthly episodes caused me serious symptoms of belly and backache, and cramps which paralysed my legs and sometimes even my arms which caused me to faint.

So, for years the first two days of menstruation totally incapacitated me! I wonder how many of you girls/ladies out there can relate to this?

The transition of girl into womanhood should be celebrated and explained clearly to little girls, so that no shame but only pride can be felt about the change. Is it any wonder then that my psoas or core muscles froze and caused the cramps?

> *Self-denial – denying my self – not allowing my own truth to show itself. So afraid of being hit or ridiculed – not allowing my self-worth to*

LESSON 1

> *develop. Constantly standing to attention and always ready to try and please her.*

In 2005 my husband, a keen Harley-Davidson enthusiast, wanted to make a mammoth trip to Nordkapp, Norway on his Harley – to celebrate his 50 years of life on earth.

I sat pillion and thus began a trip of a lifetime. We saw beautiful fjords over and over again, at a relentless 40 miles an hour, with a burning left hip joint – to the point when I nearly screamed… "Not another f . . . fjord!" We rode through towering sheets of ice in the Arctic Circle, into the one hot summer's day of Narvik, tried to crouch on the step next to a Sami lady, stood endless minutes next to the Harley before taking one step, and hauled my leg over the huge luggage pack to wedge myself between hubby and panniers!

At last in Nordkapp we stood there and I gave in! On our return to UK I would find a hip surgeon and brave the operation.

12th October 2005 Mr McMinn gave me my new shiny ball and socket in Birmingham. A hip resurfacing which took longer in the operating theatre, than for a total hip replacement, but would hopefully give me full range of movement, without the risk of dislocation. So far it is fantastic, but I had reached the point when self-denial had to change. I had to face up to a new approach to my life of exercise and towards myself.

"Six-pack Nad" had to learn the "art of softening" to help her body heal and needed to understand that it was all right to show vulnerability.

The hardness approach had broken my body, and now I needed to learn how to help it better.

Time came when I needed to remember my peers and friends in Africa, where I went to school in my teens, and how lean, supple and toned everyone seemed. How tall and proud they all walked, without the need of work-outs.

So came my next revelation! Good posture!

Positive Affirmation for arthritis:

"I am love, I now choose to love and approve of myself. I see others with love".

("Heal your Body", Louise Hay)

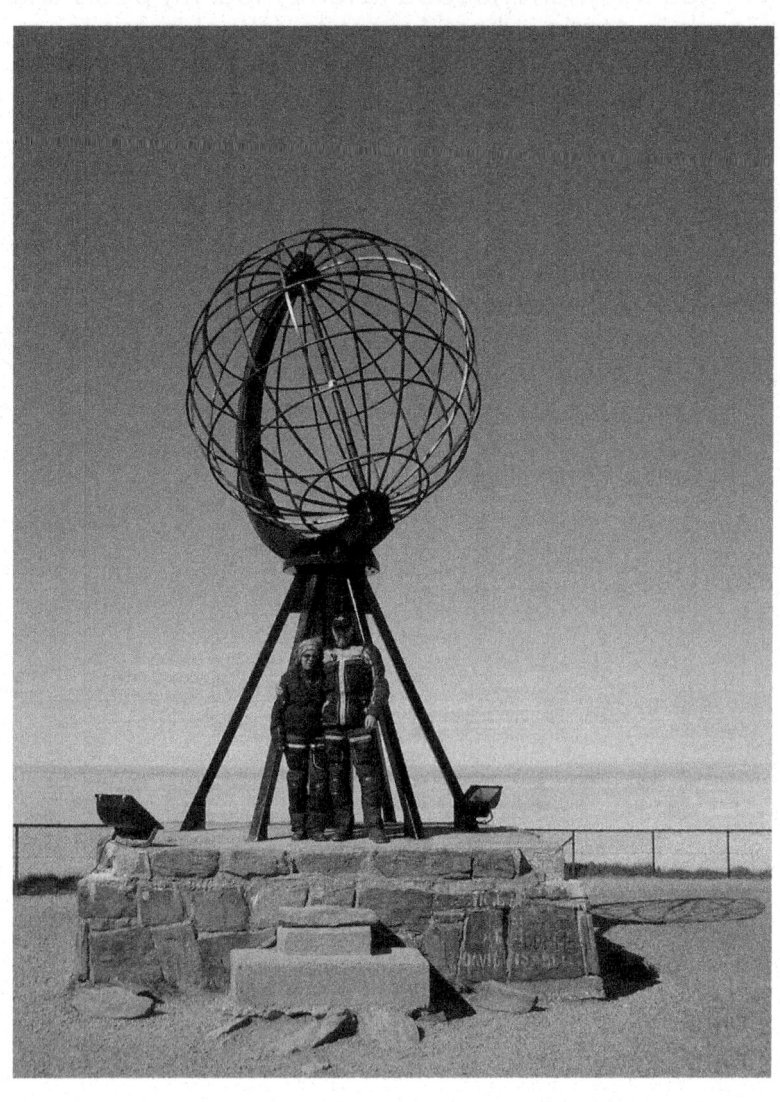

My husband Roger and I at Nordkapp, 2005

LESSON 2
GOOD POSTURE!

Joints:

> *"Represent changes in direction in life and the ease of these movements"*
>
> ("Heal your Body", Louise Hay)

LESSON 2
GOOD POSTURE!

December 2008, Canyon Country, LA.

I stayed at my youngest half-sister's house when our father passed away a few months after his 80th birthday – one year and two months after my mother's death, on 12th October 2007, in Zambia, Central Africa. They had not been together for 57 years on earth only to be re-united in spirit once again! Two peas in a pod...

Despite the sad departure of my Muslim father, who was given a grand send-off, to rest in the Eternal Valley, LA – it was another snatched moment to be with my three younger half-sisters. Bitter sweet!

Up to then my body was recovering really well from the left hip operation in 2005 (note how my mother died exactly two years onwards to the day! Was she trying to make 12th October a truly unforgettable date?).

One cold morning at my sister's house I decided to practise yoga while following a television yoga programme. It felt great that I could manage postures carefully after years of not having been able to. There was a little hindrance, however . . . this time in my right hip! A click or something . . . From that day on I gave my right hip all my attention, especially as I could eventually not cross it over my left leg without groin pain.

This time the alarm bells my body gave were not ignored, and upon my return from California a few days after my father's burial, back in England, I booked to have an X-ray.

The verdict was, it was mild to moderate arthritic deterioration, but considered normal at my age of 56! "Just stay active and if it gets too bad take painkillers". I was sent packing!!

LESSON 2

Months went by when it began to hinder my dog-walking and Qi Gong practice (Chinese Healing Movements), so I used visualization to help rebuild the worn cartilage. I asked the Universe for healing and guidance, and started to explore stem-cell regeneration.

I wanted to save my right hip naturally, without invasive surgery. The muscles in my right leg were still strong, and there was no way I would be in denial as I had been with the left leg, until the hip joint was bone on bone, and none of the muscles worked any longer. This time I learnt my lesson and the right leg became my friend. I promised I would take care of it to the best of my ability.

During this time my lower back pain was excruciating, and every time I sat down it felt as though my tail-bone was sitting on a knife's edge. Standing for any length of time was impossible, without having to accommodate the pain by leaning forward. I felt as if my lumbar back was in an iron harness.

In June, Roger (my husband) and I drove to Cologne, in Germany to the Xcell stem cell Centre, where we would meet the surgeon, who would extract bone marrow from my sitting bone (at the iliac crest), and to separate the stem cells from the marrow in order to inject them into my right hip socket, so that they could help the worn cartilage rebuild itself.

We arrived the next morning early, where we had to read the contra-indications and fill in forms, after which we seemed to wait hours for him – or that's how it seemed, which caused me to hurry to the "Ladies" rather too frequently due to nerves and fear. When he finally came to fetch me the surgeon and I walked down this shiny floored corridor into a little cell-like ante-room, where he gave me a net-like hat to wear and similar ones to cover my shoes. Then we went into the next "cell", where

Good Posture!

a pretty masked nurse was ready to assist and which also consisted of a couch and a trolley with lots of empty phials and some implements.

The surgeon re-assured me that he regularly extracted bone marrow from his own iliacus and his wife's! It sounded pretty crazy to me!

So, I was kindly instructed to lie on my front on a narrow gel covered mould type mattress and headrest on the couch, on my left side. I only needed to pull a corner of my trousers down to bare part of the iliac crest. He covered this area with sterile paper with a square cut out to narrow down the area from which to extract my bone marrow. He then sprayed some cold anaesthetic, waited a while and repeated this action once more, after which he prodded me about with a ballpoint pen, then ruffled this area with his hand. This was followed with an anaesthetic injection, another apparent "ruffle" and then he proceeded to screw, a corkscrew like implement into my sitting bone! It was not nice, nor was the endless sensation of bone marrow being sucked out. The only way I can describe it, it was as if my life force was being drained out!

He filled twenty phials with my bone marrow (a thick dark red liquid), 180ml in total! Every time he filled one phial I heard a click and then another was plugged on till all twenty were full!

After this procedure was over we then had to see the Centre's huge manager, to deal with all the paperwork and finances – a total of €7,545!

The following morning when we saw my surgeon he triumphantly told me they extracted over 7,000,000 stem cells from my bone marrow, the average, he told me was 2,000,000, so mine was "excellent!" I was ushered into

LESSON 2

an operating theatre, with a video screen above a very high couch. The surgeon sprayed on the same cold local anaesthetic onto my right outer and front part of my hip.

The longest needles and syringes appeared and were inserted at the side and then the front of the hip, all the while he looked onto the X-ray screen in order to aim these syringes into the very narrow space of my right ball and socket, to squirt my millions of stem cells into that space!

I was scared to say the least! But my amazing surgeon did it and was delirious with joy for managing to get both needles into the narrow space, and once done he did some bizarre clog dance around the operating theatre!!

Afterwards he stuck a couple of little plasters on the injected area, and I was free to walk back to my husband who was waiting in the orange and white waiting room. The whole procedure took about five to ten minutes. I had to take antibiotics for three days, but I was also self-medicating with grapefruit extract, arnica and rhus.tox, two homeopathic remedies.

The surgeon told me that cartilage regrowth takes between six weeks to three months, and that he did wish people with arthritis would come during the first stage in arthritis! So, I asked him how many stages there were to which he replied, "Four!" He told me I was in the third stage!! He hoped it would stave off new hip surgery, and give the new hip inventors a chance to invent a super duper one!! By which time I hoped I'd never need one anyway! The only problem to this is that people never tend to feel pain in the first stages of osteo-arthritis, so one wouldn't necessarily know that joint degeneration was happening!

Good Posture!

So, if you, my reader, are considering this form of treatment, check first to see what stage you are at! Simply because after this gruelling experience, and limping around the Lindt Chocolate factory, and the 4711 Cologne shop, with a weighted down hip, leaning on a walking stick, hoping this would rebuild the cartilage... well, it did not!

The German efficiency nevertheless astounded us, and the surgeon arranged for me to see a podiatrist, who within an hour, had made imprints of my foot and made me leather insoles for my shoe, there and then, in order to level out my hips, which the surgeon had measured and found that the left leg was 5 millimetres shorter than the right!

In July 2009, just a week after the German experience I did another Core Awareness course with Liz Koch. This was most valuable as she introduced us to Esther Gokhale's book, "Eight Steps to a Painfree Back". This book changed my life and eased pain that no therapist had been able to help me with.

The miracle of this was how I addressed my posture, especially when standing and walking.

My right hip still felt "sloshy" during the Application Course and my back had developed such severe lordosis that doing the simplest psoas releasing exercises was simply excruciating.

What this course emphasised to me was the importance of how my body felt at all times – how by simply applying Esther's "inner corset", which is a gentle spinal decompression, helped ease the searing lumbar ache greatly. When walking the pain eased as long as I kept focusing on decompressing my spine.

LESSON 2

Then came the memory of the proud looking women in Kenya and Zambia, carrying buckets of water, or large bundles of wood on their head, with ease, dignity and best of all straight backs.

Since the Alexander Technique approach I had become my own constant nag, whenever I walked, sat down or lay in bed. This brought such a strong inner body awareness to the foreground, making me realize that despite all my years as a Fitness Instructor I had been more concerned about my external appearance, while ignoring all the aches internally. Until I reached a point of no return.

When a colleague of mine assisted me with adductor stretches, she exclaimed how twisted my body looked! She was right! Unbeknown to me my muscles had adapted to the skeletal misaligning, and torqued around to the left, raising the left pelvic bone way higher than the right, and twisting the whole sitting bone around to the left.

No wonder my back ached constantly!

As this had been a gradual development, I had not noticed – I relied on my "strong" outer harness so much, while "gritting my teeth" and ignoring all the alarm signals from my body,

April 2011, I was due to have my right hip resurfaced. This time on the NHS, as in 2005 I had been fortunate enough to benefit from my husband's BUPA insurance and have the operation done privately!

Despite all my above-mentioned adventures at saving the right hip naturally, damage was too far gone, pain returned despite the stem cells, and adjusting my posture

Good Posture!

correctly became increasingly impossible, as all my muscles were pulling me so tightly again.

As I am a very active person and one on a mission, I sought out my NHS surgeon in an NHS hospital not so far from home, who had studied hip resurfacing with Mr McMinn himself.

I was happy for him to operate and he was with me, so I was on his list!

April 2011 was an unusually hot month here in Herefordshire and I took some rest in my hammock, providing my body with some well-earned vitamin D from the sun (all to help towards bone strength).

11th April arrived and there we were waiting to be seen by my surgeon, paper knickers on, operating gown and great felt-tip lines and crosses on my right leg – to make sure they didn't cut the other side by mistake!

I started to get a little restless and anxious, my right hip itched a lot, I thought, "mosquito bites maybe?"

By the time my surgeon came to me to take one last look to make sure I hadn't changed my mind, he looked at the place where the incision would be made . . . lo and behold there were three huge red bites, which had grown in minutes of sitting there!

The phone rings and friends are calling Roger in the car: "How's Nad?", "Is she in the operating theatre?" etc. "No", he answers," she's in the car going home! It's been postponed till next month, because of enormous horsefly bites on her bum!"

LESSON 2

May 2011 – The procedure went smoothly and from that moment onwards I was able to gently apply all the different aspects of posture, which needed to change.

January 2016 – My pelvis suddenly dropped lower, which was followed by a dramatic lengthening of back muscles and gut re-organisation, as everything is connected. From having a very lordotic back, my shape suddenly altered! And that five and a half years post-op!

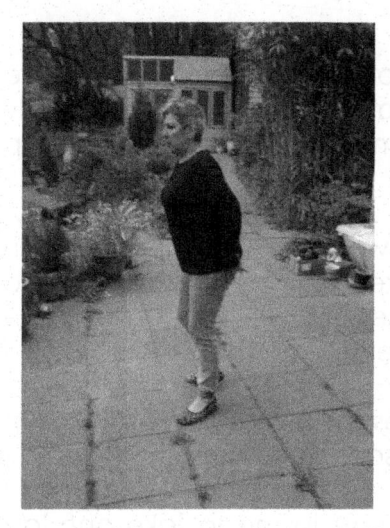

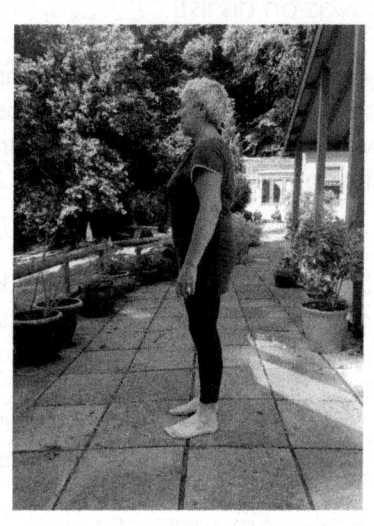

My painful pre-op stance 2011   My posture after my pelvis dropped

Why? Because I am constantly aware of keeping my spine decompressed, walking "on a line" and propelling each step from my toes, while imagining I am carrying a bucket of water on my head.

It was important to be forever conscious of my posture, as I noticed how my mother's head and neck were stuck in a forward thrusting pattern, like a turtle neck! I took it that she was my teacher, as we have similar physiques and I did not want to end up looking like that in my old age.

Good Posture!

I made a pact with myself twenty years ago that I would one day be an upright and flexible old lady. I thank my mother, Liz Koch, my African friends and the Gokhale method for this incredible transformation.

I figured that if we want to avoid osteo-arthritis and or protect our new hips, we need to change our approach to how we undertake our activities, and work together with our body so it will function to the 100% we expect it to.

The ten years from 2005 to 2015 have been enormously life changing for me, as my career was on hold twice due to the hip operations, both my parents passing away and my husband having a major career change, and who suffered years' long depression, through work dissatisfaction which we interpreted as part of the ageing process!

I have had to re-assess my direction in life and could have chosen to retire, however my hips have woken me to a calling that is stronger than myself.

They are pushing me in a direction where I am compelled to share my experience for the good of mankind, in order to help avoid pain and find the fluidity within our body, and to learn to trust our bodies fearlessly.

Positive affirmation for Joints:

> *"I easily flow with change. My life is divinely guided and I am always going in the best direction."*
>
> ("Heal your Body", by Louise Hay)

LESSON 3
CONTROL

"Hips - Carries the body in perfect balance. Major thrust in moving forward."

("Heal your Body", by Louise Hay)

Control

Ever since I can remember I always felt a force driving and protecting me, so whenever my mother punished me (which was very often!), or I was in a bad situation something in my head always reassured me and said, "You will get your reward!" So, I have always believed that, and still do, it isn't anything any human or book ever taught me.

Despite this inner knowing I still felt the need to control my own destiny, and did this by first being a tomboy in order to take care of my beautiful looking single mother – i.e. changing tyres on her Cortina GT, or replacing spark plugs! So, I created a tough image in order to cope, but all subconsciously.

In 1965 my mother and I left Belgium to return to Kenya, where my father's family lived and where he had gone to school. Not to see them, however, quite on the contrary! Mum got her new status quo as the Belgian Ambassador's personal assistant and warned me not to tell anyone that my father was Asian, as I would not have any "white" friends! She even cut my hair very short and made me look down for my passport photo, as my eyes were brown and too big, and everyone would know that I was Asian!

Fear through my mother's iron fist was by then well and truly imprinted, though as a growing child this was normal for me. I was terrified of displeasing her and was totally in awe of her throughout most of my life.

In the meantime, I retaliated by breaking as many rules at the schools I attended, while trying to cheer people up – is it any surprise that I was expelled from the three decent schools in Nairobi at that time?

LESSON 3

1979.

Our son was born and five months later he was diagnosed with Cerebral Palsy, and I was told he may never walk!

Something I never really wanted to talk about is the fact that our little 5-month old son was diagnosed with Cerebral Palsy in early 1980. I realise, however, the strength of impact this has had on both my husband's and my life.

We had just begun our lives as a young adventurous little threesome out in the Central African bush of Zambia, where Roger took his first overseas teaching contract at 24 years of age. As a young family, we were warned during a week's briefing about our new life in the bush at Farnham Castle, about the hazards of accompanying wives becoming "excess luggage"! The possibilities of boredom driving them to becoming alcoholics and suffering from neurosis! Fat chance of that happening to me!

Our first month there, we had to make a home out of a very dirty house on the compound, after which I set out to teach myself how to cook, make my own crafts, sew and be a mummy! We had a lucky star shining on us, however, as within our first day there we met a wonderful Norwegian family with two small children, who had lived on the compound for nearly three years by then, and who had got a great survival system and shopping strategy sorted out! They taught us all we needed to know and more. They were both teachers at the same school where Roger worked, and although their contract lasted for another six months, we have remained life-long friends till this day. We had wonderful adventures together and went on safaris, and they were of tremendous support to us.

Control

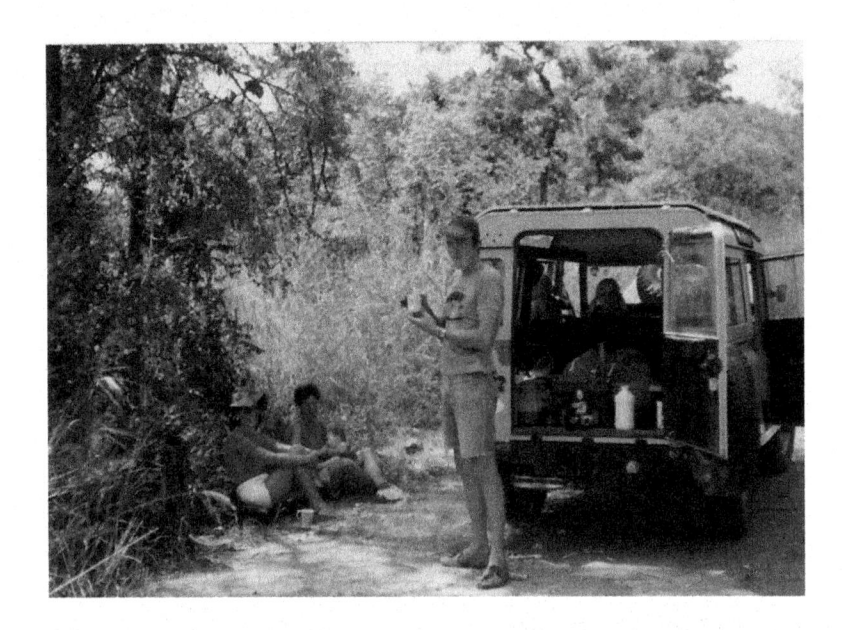

On safari with our Norwegian friends in Zambia, 1980

Our blissful and exciting first month was short-lived as our baby developed infantile spasms, a form of epilepsy. I returned to the UK by the end of that first month in Africa, with our little one to get treatment and medication. That is when our world shattered when receiving his diagnosis.

For the next seven years I became his full-time occupational and physiotherapist, and delved into my creative vault to find ways of stimulating our adorable and jolly little boy. To help him gain some sense of balance when sitting, to see and focus on objects and us from a distance, to get him out of his long blank spells when he seemed to wander off into another "dimension".

My job as "excess luggage" was cut out for me and I embraced it with love and joy and a real drive. I learned how to become wife/mother/cook/therapist during those six years in Zambia. We adored our little boy, so this was a challenge we faced together and Roger learned

LESSON 3

to be a real handyman and carpenter. He built our boy walkers, standing frames and corner seats. He became an adept Landrover mechanic, electrician and all-round protector. We both learned the skills of self-sufficiency and adaptation to the various circumstances which offered themselves to us.

1982.

Our second little son was born while out in Eastern province of Zambia. He was very premature, at 28 weeks, born at the nearest mission hospital 20 miles from where we lived. He popped out so quickly, unlike our first boy who took three days, and who was born at 36 weeks. This little one cried, and was very much alive, but still waxy and didn't look "quite ready". He was whisked away from me and put in a little wooden box surrounded by hot-water bottles. Roger kept the heaters on full blast in the Landrover as our baby had to be rushed to another bigger mission hospital 56 miles further, where they had incubators. Our German nurse friend who held my hand during the birth, decided it was better for the baby to hold him against her skin during the long journey, which is what she did. I was told by the midwife Sister to stay behind to be looked after!

The next day my hubby drove me to be with my little baby, and when we arrived the exhausted European doctor/midwife, who had been on duty for over 72 hours without sleep, told us they'd had to resuscitate Laurie (we gave him a name of course!) already twice.

That day and night I spent either wandering around helplessly in the cattle-shed type ward, with wind howling through, wafting smells of cabbage all around us, and visiting my little boy in his starched hospital gown inside the incubator, with cockroaches running around inside it. The other pass-time was joining the group of Zambian

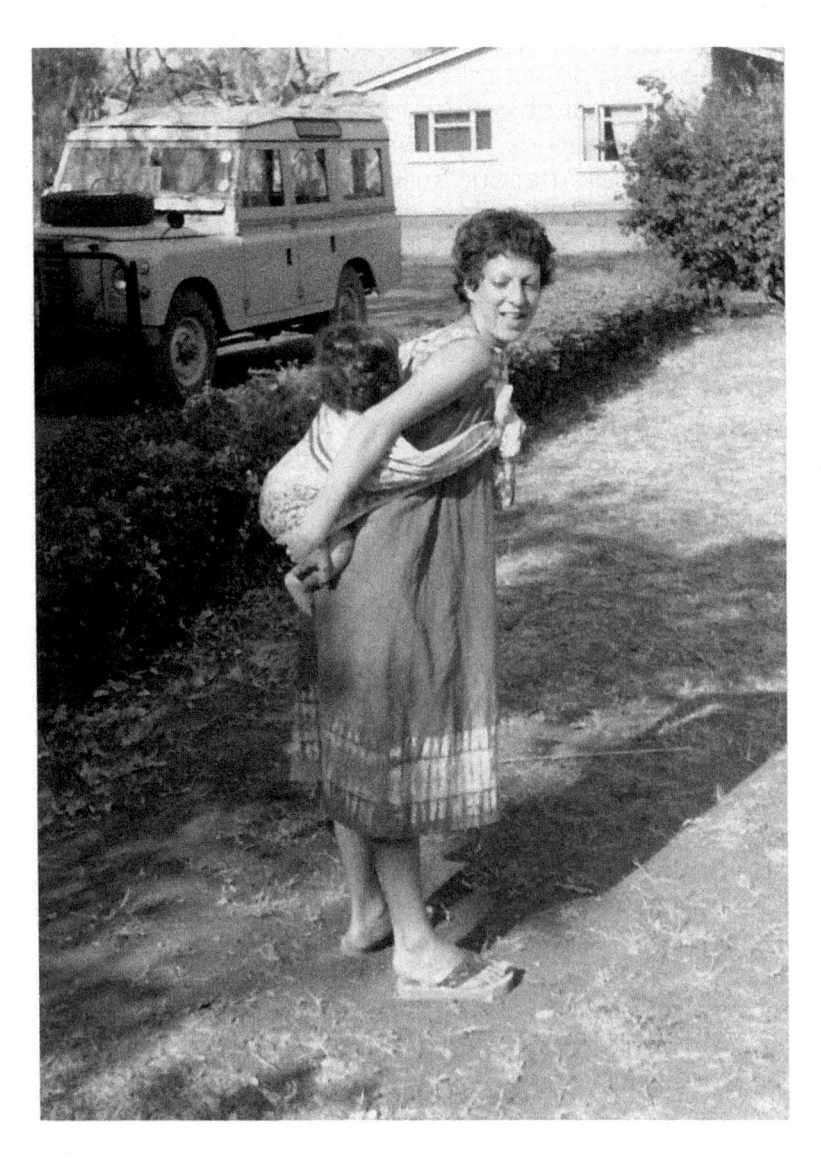

At home on the Teacher's Compound,
Petauke Secondary School, Zambia. 1980

LESSON 3

young mothers in a communal room where we sat in a circle expressing our milk by hand. All I could contribute was a tiny bit of colostrum to add to the rich milk these ladies produced as they were still breastfeeding their previous child! After our "milking session" we then had to pour our contribution in a common green plastic bowl, which would then be used to feed the premature babies!

Three days after our baby's birth they had one final attempt at resuscitating him, when he decided that this earth life was not for him, and so he returned to his original home.

The African staff were very sweet and philosophical, they shook our hands good-bye, and advised us to go home and make another baby!

Now there is a lonesome little grave under an acacia tree, with a home-made cross with its branches, in Katete Mission Hospital. Laurie's spirit is free; however, he gave us the opportunity to truly focus on his older little brother.

We returned to our compound home to digest all that had happened so quickly, and felt shell-shocked. I spent hours sitting under our mango tree grieving the loss of Laurie, my body feeling cheated as I was now producing huge amounts of milk, but with no baby to feed. The young Dutch doctor at the mission hospital apologetically gave me the only drug he could obtain to dry my milk production, which made me put on loads of weight quickly, as I was really thin in those days.

Thankfully, our three-year old son kept us sane and filled our days with love and laughter. We had also employed a wonderful Zambian lady to be his nanny during my pregnancy, as lifting my 3-year old, who could not walk became a little strenuous, and she was a Godsend!

In the meantime, we continued to gain experiences on survival, as within the first year of our life in the Eastern Province of Zambia, the water stopped flowing. My new vegetable garden dried out and we programmed ourselves to wake up at 3AM, to swap the hosepipe from one full white-painted dustbin to fill the other with the trickle of water which is all that reached us at that time of day! So, water was rationed and this situation became a bit of a nightmare with regards to boiling nappies! No such thing as disposables! Bath water was recycled and we kept a paddling pool with water to have a "shower" in!

Every two months we would travel at the crack of dawn to the Eastern province capital, Chipata, to go to the market. That was an entire expedition in itself, as we needed to prepare in case of a breakdown with the Landrover and carry jerry cans of petrol, water, take food, drink and blankets, as we were travelling through desolate bush with few clusters of mud huts along the way. Of course these were the pre-mobile phone days!

We arrived at the bustling market at around 7-8AM, after a three-hour journey, to stock up with fresh vegetables, fruit and meat, all commodities which were rare in our village. This trip always turned into a special treat, as we would go and have a curry in one of the local restaurants, not always guaranteed to be safe on our stomachs!

Then followed the long trip back home, and of course with our little one, who accompanied us everywhere. Once home and he was safely tucked in his cot, we spent several hours blanching and freezing our fresh supplies, and butchering the meat, in order to have food for the next two months.

Our little local supermarket in the Boma (the village centre), had mainly empty shelves, and mostly stocked

LESSON 3

ominous looking coloured squash, called Jolly Juice. Cooking oil, sugar, flour were rare commodities and no sooner as the lorry arrived in the Boma, everybody would rush to the supermarket to stand in queues for hours to buy their rations. We would get a 25Kg bag of flour, which I would then bag up in smaller quantities and freeze, and the rest would stay in the sack, to be sieved in order to get rid of the weevils, before making bread! During bread-making days I also made pizzas, which we would eat that day, and then freeze the rest. Everything we wanted we had to make ourselves, including tomato ketchup!

We also employed a house-boy, called James, whom I taught to cook basic meals and bake our bread. He was worth his weight in gold! Both he and Nanny stayed with us for the six years we lived in Africa. We needed their help as there were no washing machines, and I spent all day either preparing food in advance, occupying my baby, making crafts, curtains, clothes . . .

Very often we went weeks without electricity, so then we learned from both of them how to use the local charcoal fires, which were cylindrical shaped and the size of a large paint pot. Once I cooked food for 36 people on two of those! Whenever we had a power cut for more than three days, we would cook the entire contents of the freezer and have a party for our local friends! It was a great excuse to socialize!

This is how as a young family we learned to be self-sufficient, how survival's necessities helped us cope with the loss of our second little boy and how it made us question our purpose on this earth.

We moved for the last three years in Central Africa to the southern province of Zambia to my mother's farmhouse, by the Zambezi River, which set the new pattern of me becoming a fitness instructor, and amateur artist.

1986.

We returned to England, after those momentous six years in Zambia. Roger's contract ended and he didn't want to renew it, moreover we needed to find new ways of helping our 6-year old son.

Circumstances and deep heartache forced us to deal with these challenges to the best of our abilities. We both were given a book by a friend while in Zambia, "Out on a Limb", by Shirley MacLaine, which created a huge shift within both of us, and helped open our eyes to spirituality and our purpose.

It was during 1982-83 that I became a devout… Fitness fanatic and instructor, creating a real stir in Livingstone, Southern Province, Zambia, for three years, while putting big groups of people through their paces to terrific music.

So, the pattern was set as far as my physical activities were concerned and I became ultra-fit!

On our return to UK, and after one year of our little 6-year old son attending a special school, he regressed physically; I took him out of school, with the headmistress' blessing. Thus began our journey of intensive alternative therapies to help improve his quality of life.

We travelled to Hungary, the Ukraine, took him to hyperbaric oxygen chambers, had his gym built, worked with an army of volunteers, and fund raised endlessly.

Some external force seemed to drive me again, and although everything we wanted always came our way regarding our boy and therapies, I was like a manic woman on a mission.

LESSON 3

Fighting with authorities, pushing to get him accepted here and there, and as our son put it one day, "My mum will fight like a little tiger to get me accepted!"

So life happened, dear reader, which will probably be familiar to you, though your circumstances differ. One way or another we always try to control our destiny, not giving this Universal Force, call it God, Allah, the Source or whatever suits you best, a chance to assist us.

Then when my colleague told me that my body was twisted, as I mentioned in Lesson 2, it really halted me in my track. I had lost touch with myself!

I had been so busy trying to control change in my son's life, and prove the doctors wrong, that my son would walk at the cost of what I was doing to myself. I thought I was infallible! Of course, "I can cope, my aerobic classes were keeping me strong!" I thought!

Change.

Then, Change, happened – time for our son to start school! Later than most children, but we found a great school with Hungarian therapists (called Conductors), who would continue his exercises.

My husband commuted to work daily, and suddenly my life seemed to come to a standstill. I felt as though my purpose for living, and that which drove me, had been snatched away from me, and for the first time in a long time, I felt so alone. I lost my direction! According to Louise Hay's little book "Heal your body", the hips carry the body forward, especially when new decisions are to be made.

I was afraid of change and from then onward all the physical pain came to the foreground. My hips and back started to scream at me, "Stop now! Take care of me – if you do we will work as a perfect team!"

Did I take notice of the alarm bells my hips and back were ringing? Of course not!

The rest of the story you already know!

Really the reason I share part of this journey with you is in order to help you perhaps see more clearly what patterns occur in your life, which may relate to mine, but through different circumstances, of course.

I felt I had nothing to move forward to, which relates totally with what Louise Hay describes.

Then on one of my aimless days I watched a programme on TV about the neglect of disabled Romanian orphans. As I was sitting on the settee, I suddenly felt as if there was a gentle earthquake! Then I realised it was my body vibrating like an electric wire, and I couldn't stop it. It seemed to last for ages, and when I stood up and touched the wall, it was as if the whole house was live!

Some force seemed to drive through me giving me an electrical surge, and an irrepressible desire to serve mankind. I felt I must do something important, but had no idea what!

It was at that time that despite still being a Fitness instructor, since 1990 I had also started practising Qi Gong – Chinese Healing movements, which is a totally different approach to Western health and fitness. It is an art which accesses and cultivates internal energy rather than expending it. So, it was this gentle practice which assisted in my gradual softening and trusting more in the

LESSON 3

natural state of being, one which as a growing child I had always observed from my African peers, who were always cheerful and happy, despite having very little material wealth.

My angry outbursts, which were always directed at my poor hubby, calmed down and the hip issues really came to the foreground.

The best thing of all is that it taught me to shut "the drunken monkey chatter" in my brain off. This I did by using a medium's visualization, giving my busy mind something else to focus on for a short while.

The "drunken monkey" which was always telling me how to control situations started to become quieter. Do you know what happened then? It gave this Universal Force, Source, God, Allah, Angels, Guides, however you wish to call it, a chance to give me Peace!

I started to feel a serene type of stillness, which gradually made space in my busy mind, for "New Ideas" to enter, for new insights and a calmness I had rarely experienced before in my life.

This started me off on my new journey of insight and trust!

Positive affirmation for hips:

"Hip hip hooray – there is joy in every day, I am balanced and free."

("Heal your body", by Louise Hay)

LESSON 4
TRUST

Hips:

"Fear of going forward in major decisions. Nothing to move forward to"

("Heal your body" by Louise Hay)

LESSON 4
TRUST

In 2001 I met my Grandmaster Yang Mei Jun, the amazing Wild Goose Qi Gong Inheritor, at 105 years of age. The meeting happened in Beijing, China, where I was to observe Tui Na and Qi Gong doctors at work in the Xi Yuan University Hospital for three weeks. The meeting with Grandmaster was amazing and happened with incredible ease, as if this was pre-ordained. We drove by taxi through a wintry snow and ice-covered Beijing. I was accompanied by another lady on the course and our Chinese taxi driver who with his smattering of English was going to be my interpreter. It was with enormous trepidation that we walked upstairs to the first floor of her apartment, and we were welcomed by her student, who took care of her.

We were invited into the dining area and served lovely tea, then her strong loud voice beckoned us to her room where she was sitting on her little bed. She wore a beautiful deep red satin jacket, and a woollen bobble hat. Both my friend and I felt we had entered a very special shrine.

I kneeled beside her and held her hand, and for quite some time Grandmaster Yang Mei Jun stared at my heart area – or middle Dan Tien (Crystal Field), and suddenly I felt the entire heart area start to spin slowly, like a vortex, or more a washing machine! It was such a real and physical sensation that I was convinced my friend could see it happening. She was dumbfounded and in awe of being in this powerful lady's presence. We both were.

Till this day I am grateful for this stunning encounter and for weeks afterwards, back in England I was buzzing again like a live electric wire. There was a reason why we met and thank goodness that I did, as she passed away the next year.

LESSON 4

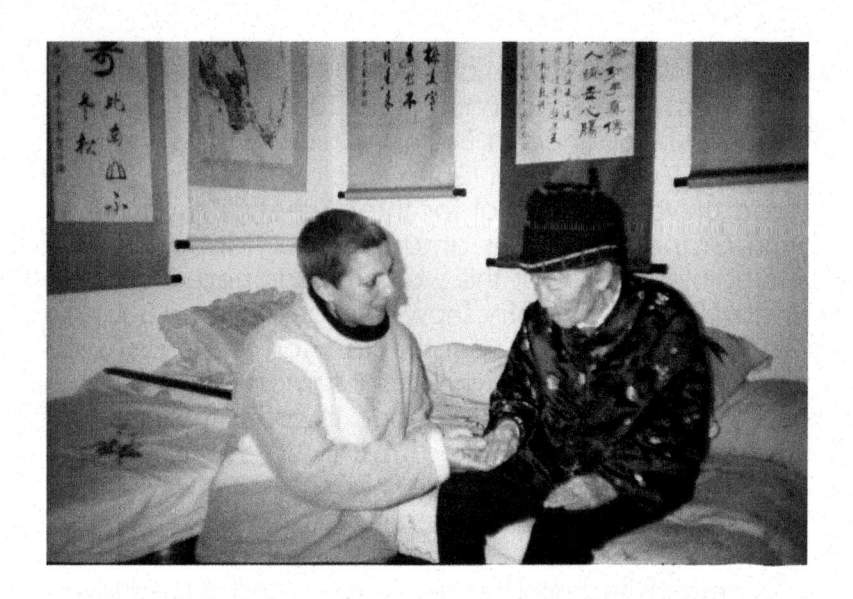

Grandmaster Yang Mei Jun and me, Beijing 2001

Our connection was sealed and ever since we met I very much feel guided by her spirit, which has urged me to develop a very natural form of Qi Gong (Chi Kung) – one with no form, but which comes from within each and every one of us. One which activates our own individual movements' choreographer, simply by connecting to our fluids and the "universal chiropractor"!

Starting to connect with this part of my being involved deep trust and one which told my "control tower" to hush, so the mind could take a back seat, while letting the body do its random "somatic" movements.

This was no coincidence, as already for a few years I had been teaching some Qi Gong forms, but was never happy to do so. The reason for this was that Qi Gong's essence is to heal, and yet the pain I felt never abated, quite the contrary it got worse.

This helped me reach the conclusion that no matter how gentle the disciplined exercise is, when we have an unknown injury, it can aggravate it. Allowing the body to move instinctively, however, gives it the opportunity to soften, release the tension, help the blood to flow where it was stuck and heal itself.

Goodness, what a miraculous discovery and how it really puts into place the true essence of Qi Gong. This very powerful self-healing system, which has been used since time immemorial – well before some clever people decided to share their discoveries by giving the natural movements form!

Thus, True to our Roots Qi Gong was born! At once I regained my purpose and ability to move forward in my life, and therefore also the ability to undo the initial problems which caused osteo-arthritis in the first place.

> "You are not your history; you are who you choose to be" (Carl Jung).

My suggestion to you, dear reader is to look into your past and retrace the years to find what happened to you primarily, to have given you, for example low self-esteem or self-worth. Who were the first people in your life who may have criticised you, or didn't show you the love any small child needs and deserves? Then begin to undo these negative issues by learning to look at yourself in the mirror with love rather than dislike or hatred. Louise Hay's book "You Can Heal Your Life" will give you a wonderful insight on how to begin to heal your own life.

As a result of my own personal detective work at self-realization I have come across several self-healing methods. One very powerful method which can happen involuntarily during spontaneous Qi Gong is shaking. The latter's physiological phenomenon is one we have learned to suppress in order to survive in our pressing society and culture. What we have learnt to do very cleverly is suppress the expression of fear as much as we can as a coping mechanism. This is unnatural to us and all mammals, and our reptilian or involuntary "background operating system", which keeps all our basic functions, organs, blood-flow etc. ticking away, has helped us to freeze our emotions – if you can't fight or run away, you freeze. This unfortunately is very counterproductive for us, as that unexpressed fear manifests itself in different ways: irrational thinking, behaviour or emotions, such as Post Traumatic Stress Disorder, illness, aches and pains. If unaddressed these symptoms can become life threatening dis-eases in later life.

David Berceli, founder of TRE (Trauma Release Exercises, author of "The Revolutionary Trauma Release Process" book and others) has devised a series of exercises which activate the core muscles to help trigger off our shaking mechanism, which in turn alleviates layer upon layer of deeply held tension, trauma and stress from the body's central nervous system. He has been using this phenomenal method to help thousands of people in war-torn and poverty-stricken countries, in order to help them cope better with their daily stresses and strains.

If we relearn this ancient and natural method and use it as a form of relaxation in our busy lives, we then take charge once again of our own health and well-being.

The shaking can lead into our wonderful fascial (our connective tissue) lubrication and involuntary stretches and movements, which I call Spontaneous Qi Gong, and Emily Conrad's Continuum Movements (founder and author of "Life on Land").

I was fortunate enough to attend Emily's three-day workshop in London in June 2013, where amongst others, she singled me out, and put me on the stage as a guinea-pig with two metal hips. We made a beautiful connection, and at some point she stood in front of me, while I had been submerged in my own spontaneous fluid movement, and she told me "I love the way you work!" That was music to my ears, and confirmation by the Master of fluid movement (Emily had been developing Continuum Movement for over forty years), that I was doing something right!

I excitedly looked forward to her second trip to UK in 2014, when to my shock and horror she died in April 2014, just before her eightieth year!

So, yet another wonderful movement "Master" I was fated to meet fleetingly, but forever memorable.

Now Grandmaster Yang Mei Jun is my "Grandma in Spirit" and Emily Conrad my "mother in spirit"! I am very fortunate to feel their energy guiding and supporting me in True to our Roots Qi Gong's development.

I feel we are connected to the entire universe. If we had no fear of death we could truly enjoy our life on earth, and make it a joyful and happy adventure, by embracing our "spirit" or "soul" and merging it with our material self.

Fear leads us into irrational behaviour, which is in the main counter-productive to ourselves only. If we could actually turn our lives on earth as our lives "in heaven", we would benefit and could be living by example on how to trust and find our joy and love while here.

Here are just a few simple methods I have come across to share with you, dear reader, on how to release the fear from your body, to learn to trust and believe in yourself and to love who you truly are. Learning to become aware

LESSON 4

of your body's sensations and posture, while going about your daily activities, and feeling the ecstasy of immersing yourself in your own healing fluids. Becoming familiar with how a delicious stretch feels when allowing the "Clingfilm effect" or fascial stretches to occur. By looking into the mirror and simply telling yourself "I love you"!

Positive affirmation for hips:

"I am in perfect balance. I move forward in life with ease and with joy at every age"

("Heal your Body" by Louise Hay)

LESSON 5
MY MOTHER'S DEATH

My Mother's Death

Taken from my blog written on 14th October 2016

Nine years ago today, a heavenly number according to the Taoist philosophy, was the day mum dropped dead! Actually, she keeled over on her settee in the sitting room in the early hours of the morning.

She stopped going to bed to sleep as she was defying death, actually she was terrified of it! So, she had put her sleeping bag on her settee with a pillow covered in a brown pillowcase, so it looked more like an ornamental cushion, and she would sit bolt upright with her dainty feet in fluffy slippers on a little grass pouffe. She would throw an old crocheted holey shawl over her shoulders as her only comfort while waiting for dawn to break. Sadly, today nine years ago dawn came when death defied her!

This intrepid and adventurous traveller was on her final journey home, after years of trying to control all and sundry who came under her rule . . . The "little empress"! Commanding her staff till the night before her departure and as her lovely "earth angel" Florence, mum's Zambian house girl wrote in her text to me yesterday:

> ". . . It was this time when mum kept on sending me out to buy milk, bananas and Whiskas . . . little did I know that I would find her gone the following day. Days fly! It's candle lighting as we continue celebrating her life as a role model. Flossie."

For the last three years of mum's life Florence became mum's daytime companion and general "dog's body". She is a very caring woman in her forties, who is Chief Mukuni's niece and also his daughter in law. He is the Chief of the Toka Leya people of the Southern Province in

LESSON 5

Zambia. After mum's passing she gave birth to a second little girl and named her after my mother!

My mother's exit from her house was how she would have wanted it. Florence ran a few kilometres across Livingstone to fetch the lady who did her meals on wheels, who then drove in her nightie with Flossie to fetch the missionary lady who was the appointed executor of mum's will. Together they drove in the latter's pick-up truck with the spare house keys back to my mother's house.

I can only imagine the chaos and the wailing which will have gone on once they were with mum! The Jamaican lady, who did the meals on wheels, grabbed the lacy oblong table cloth on the television to tie around mum's jaw, when she heard her spirit tell her to "phone Nadia!" (which she did!) By this time the lady assistant manager of the security watchmen company was there too, and together these lovely ladies carried mum on her sleeping bag out into the scorching Zambian sun and gently laid her in the back of the pick-up. Then one of the women ran back to the house to fetch her pillow to put under her head.

The missionary lady had already buried a son and her husband and thought it best to recycle their coffin, so mum was kept in a third-hand coffin in the hut mortuary near to the Livingstone hospital one street away.

We needed to organize our journey from UK to arrive there four days later, which was the quickest journey available. In the meantime mum's handy man from Sierra Leone had to constantly repair the freezer in the mortuary which kept breaking down. Organizing our journey to Livingstone was very convoluted as there was no direct flight, so we ended up flying from London to Nairobi, Kenya (where mum's and my life together in

Africa started), from there we flew to Harare, Zimbabwe, then to Lusaka, the capital of Zambia, where we waited 12 hours before taking our final connection of two hours to Livingstone in a small domestic aeroplane. This was really putting all our trust in the universe, as first of all they nearly took off without refuelling, then once ready to board, the other eight passengers rushed to get in and we realized too late why, as we ended up sitting in the tail end with seats that swivelled and wobbled and where the plane was so narrow making sitting for a big man like my husband rather squashed and uncomfortable. The advantage of such a small plane was that we could see the two Zambian pilots in their cockpit and out of the windows while they were aiming the landing strategy between rows of little white lights in the pitch black of the African night!

We were welcomed by two friends late that evening in an empty little airport, with mum's ghost standing behind the baggage reclaim with her camera in hand taking photos of her little family arriving, probably to hide the burning tears!

Our friends drove us to 87 Mambo Way, Livingstone where the dimly lit gate was opened by a paralytic drunken old Charles, the night watchman! When his bloodshot eyes recognized us, he sobbed hysterically hiding his toothless mouth in a dirty old rag.

Mum's house was steeped in an eery silence and darkness, despite her two parrots and five cats. We unlocked the padlocked chains from the wrought iron burglar gates which protected the French double doors on the front verandah.

My mother had warned me not to interfere in her household, only three months earlier when we visited her, so I felt a bit like a burglar walking into her house without

LESSON 5

her there! The reality of her not being there suddenly hit me! Once we switched the lights on and checked on the parrots and cats, our friends left and there we were making up our bed, after checking for deadly looking spiders and other creepy crawlies!

It all seemed surreal! The moment I dreaded the most in my life had dawned on me, especially as I was the only one who could sort out my mother's affairs, unlock her bedroom with all her riches, and the office with all her secrets, and 69 old-fashioned cloudy grey and white box files filled with her memories of days gone by. Her entire life was kept on paper - her travels, her career, her properties, her research into her adopted Russian father's history, her angry letters and disputes, my letters to her from when I first could write, even photos of a dead cousin and her mother on her death bed. I found her secret correspondence with my father whom she had divorced 49 years previously, but with whom she had rekindled a friendship unbeknown to any of us . . . and so much more!

The next morning Florence arrived and stood sobbing loudly in the corridor next to the kitchen. We hugged and cried together in stupefied shock at what had occurred, both heavily conscious at the huge impact this would have on both of our lives!

I mentioned before that my mother had been an adventurous and intrepid explorer - she travelled the globe fearlessly, mainly by ship or by car. Not quite the way most of us would contemplate moving from one country to another! Oh no, lock, stock and barrel, mum's final move from me was with her entire household including my grandparent's giant antique cuckoo clock, her car, her pets - everything. I stood on Southampton docks waving my home and mother away after my little offering of a net of fresh fruit for in her cabin. I was 22 and I guess she thought her job as responsible mother had ended. Thus, began her lonesome adventure as a teacher in West Africa.

The next time I saw her again was two years later, when she drove her dormobile van, after a sea journey from West Africa to Greece, all the way through Albania and the rest of Europe back to UK, in the pit of winter, through ice and snow with a van load of birds and parrots. Upon her arrival in London she parked in the underground carpark of the Overseas Development Administration buildings, until she found digs in Carshalton and a temporary teaching job. She made the headlines of the local London papers!

Mum's restless spirit took her off to Zambia a year or so later as she could not settle in the UK. That is where she stayed till the last day of her life!

She eventually became the owner of a beautiful 60-acre property on the banks of the Zambezi River, where she dreamt of creating a tourist lodge long before the first ones ever existed! Unfortunately, she did not possess the appropriate managerial skills to fulfil her dream in her "little corner of paradise", as she named it, and sadly ended up selling it after having lived there for twenty years and moved to Livingstone town.

She suffered all types of undiagnosed tropical illnesses which made living in the bush particularly difficult for this ageing little lady, and impractical. Alexandra Fuller describes mum very aptly in her book "Leaving before the Rains Come",

> . . . Grand-mere, she had asked me to call her . . . she was ending her life alone on a bend of the Zambezi River, her body flooded with an array of known and unknowable parasites.

LESSON 5

> *Her skin was yellow and she felt cold most of the time. More or less permanent malaria had thinned her blood to a watery chill. She kept a fire stoked in her bedroom, even in steaming midsummer, and at night she warmed her feet in tubs of river water brought to a boil over a fire in the kitchen. Dust and smoke covered everything she owned: a portrait of herself as a young woman in Brugge; books and maps and letters; a cuckoo clock that had long ceased working . . ."*

After Florence's hug, life became so surreal for us both and we continued to follow through what mum had put in place, like how much food the cats and parrots needed, still doing up the servants' quarters or the "kaya" into a guesthouse for the forthcoming arrival of two Japanese female volunteers, who arrived that very week.

We were grateful for all the preparatory work, which we carried out with great zeal as though it was still so important to please mum, but also to stop the process of too much thinking!

Having the volunteers stay on the premises was a god-sent for us, as it meant ongoing employment for Florence and Kachele, the garden boy, and my peace of mind whenever I returned to UK.

The next day after our arrival we had the executer of the will together with her lawyer visit us to discuss mum's will, and later on two Indian men whom we vaguely remembered from when we lived in Zambia, who came to offer their services with mum's final laying out.

That day we went to the little mortuary, which was slightly more sophisticated than a mud hut, and built from concrete blocks and mortar. Her coffin was pulled out and there she lay, under a white sheet. I was wedged between two wailing women, Florence and Melody (the meals on wheels woman), who were pulling and nudging me along through the narrow space between the coffin and the wall. I felt as though I was being bulldozed down by a fast-moving train, I could even hear it! There lay the person who had been my entire world for the first twenty-one years of my life . . . lifeless, cold with a wrinkle-free face with mouth turned down at the corners symbolising her total disillusionment with life on earth.

I wonder how she'd have coped with the thought of having to be laid out by an Indian man, after spending thirty-eight years and more, denying to all and sundry that her daughter was the product of her love affair with a handsome man from the Punjab? Instead making everyone believe that I was her first English husband's daughter!! The man who refused to divorce her as he loved her and to convince him she employed a detective to photograph her and my father in bed together, so she had grounds for divorce!

Her funeral would be within two days of our arrival and she had requested to be cremated the only way it was done in Livingstone, the Indian way, on a pyre!

I cut some of her bougainvillea flowers, and made a little bouquet to put between her hands, and gave the man one of mum's favourite caftan dresses to wear. I let my husband accompany the tiny crowd of mourners to the crematorium wasteland!

No way could I face up to watching them pour ghee (butter oil) all over her and set fire to my mother! I stayed at her house and prepared for the people to return for a cup of tea, and the non-stop supply of sandwiches and cake being brought over by Melody's driver! Until this day my husband never told me what he witnessed and I thank him for his discretion.

LESSON 5

We had strict instructions from my mother's will that her ashes should return to Belgium where she wanted to join those of our Spanish nanny, who had been a mother figure to her and the most adorable grandmother to me and my cousins.

We were advised to wait forty-eight hours before going to this crematorium to collect her ashes. There was nothing sophisticated or even sacred about the collection of mum's ashes. First, we walked to the local crafts-market and looked for a couple of carved wooden pots with lids to serve as urns, then I collected two new plastic sandwich bags from mum's kitchen drawer to fit into these pots and off we drove to the crematorium.

I knew how desolate it looked from the road, but was totally unprepared for what was in store for me. We drove through the gate in the low concrete wall surrounding a vast piece of sandy and dry wasteland on which stood a lonesome construction with a corrugated roof, under which was a little rail for the pyre carriage. Once alight it then gets pushed through an opening in the one back wall, where the body is left to burn. We walked around that wall to find the little carriage on its rails with mum's skeleton depicted in the ashes below it! Now what? We looked around and found a big spade (I had not thought I would need to do this for myself!) and gently shovelled up some of her ashes to carefully aim it into these two sandwich bags while making sure it'd all fit into these two carved pots. I wonder if mum had a chuckle then, giving me this final challenge?

We finally drove away having taken as much of the ashes as we could possibly fit in and left the rest of her to mingle with the others and the red soil of Africa she had loved so much!

One pot I decided would reside below her previous residence by the Zambezi River, her little corner of paradise, Quiet Waters, now The River Club, whose little boat we needed to place the urn in said place and we also sprinkled some of her ashes in the Zambezi River for perpetuity . . .

The bigger pot wended its way back to Belgium according to her wish!

Interestingly the day she was placed next to our Nanny, Florence had a dream. She went to mum's house while eating an ice cream cone (where she was still working), and old Charles (not drunk this time!), told her at the gate: "Madam is in the house!" Florence replied: "This can't be . . .", when she heard mum's footsteps come to the French doors and opening the doors mum said to Florence: "I'm home now, come give me that ice cream!"

Unbeknown to Florence, at that very time, during the wake my uncle in Belgium offered us ice cream to eat!

The two years following this event I spent revisiting mum's house and sorting out her entire estate, tenants, staff and pets!

What saw me through this was my relentless trust and communion with my spirit and the angelic world. It strengthened my belief that we are definitely not alone on this earth-plane. I constantly asked my guardian angel to find the appropriate angel or guide (i.e. an Estate Angel!), to assist me in fulfilling mum's will and also in clearing her entire history and part of mine in the best and most considerate way.

LESSON 5

I had moments of utter desolation, rage, sadness, but having said this I grieved for my mother years before she passed at her choice of such a lonely and virtual friendless existence. She lived with the ghosts of her past, holding on to deep unexpressed anger and regrets, and chose her material wealth and "stuff" over her little family who were there to embrace her, if only she had allowed it!

My mother was such a powerful teacher for me, and I thank her for all that she suffered in order to teach me how NOT to go about things in life, to embrace love for others as well as self, without the constant judgements and criticism. I came across these six words in one of mum's diaries: "Mea culpa, mea culpa, mea culpa . . .!" (I am guilty . . .). She tortured herself with her past memories and died a loveless, lonely little old lady whose emotional bitterness was etched over her entire being. The self-hatred surprising Florence as she was told to cover all the mirrors in the house with sheets, because she no longer saw the beauty she had once been . . .

May your spirit soar now Mum and feel the freedom, unconditional love, joy and peace back in our true home . . . thank you for all you have taught me.

I love you.

LESSON 6
TRUE TO OUR ROOTS: EXTERNAL EXERCISE VERSUS INTERNAL EXERCISE!

LESSON 6

True To Our Roots: External Exercise Versus Internal Exercise!

A new insight, yet to be digested!

When I was a fitness instructor teaching gruelling high and hard impact aerobics, (I was regarded as such a tough teacher that a big guy who was captain of a local rugby team, asked me to give them physical training sessions!), I also started to incorporate the gentle Qi Gong forms into my daily practice and a state of confusion started to arise within my psyche! What was best for me? Western keep fit which gave me a high, or Eastern Qi Gong which made me calm?

A Chinese Qi Gong doctor asked me once why I was still teaching aerobics while in my forties. He pointed to the fish-bellies of my hands, which connect to the lung meridians and said: "Your lungs are depleted; you should just practise Qi Gong and replenish your heart and lungs Qi or energy, or you will die prematurely!!

His words stayed engrained with me until now, when I can at long last share them with you with a much deeper understanding. The words which will follow may really rock your belief system, but they come from an internal place of wisdom as I understand my body and energy system so much better.

According to Traditional Chinese Medicine based on the 6,000 years old Taoist philosophy of how "we are all moving forward along the path of life, gathering a greater understanding, longevity and spiritual development:

> *"When you do external exercise*
> *you must do internal exercise*
> *When you do internal exercise*
> *you may forget to do external exercise."*

LESSON 6

> (Excerpt taken from Dr Stephen Chang's book "The complete system of self-healing internal exercises".)

So in Traditional Chinese Medicine we learn that our energy or Qi courses through channels or meridians (like blood does through our veins and arteries), of which the main 12 channels are connected to our internal organs.

When we learn to allow our body to do its own fluid stretches, giving us an instant feel-good factor, and once you know these channels or meridians run along the full length of your body, legs, feet, arms, hands, then you will understand that our natural stretches, which vary from individual to individual are actually clearing blocked energy and helping to re-harmonise our internal organs. Our bodies have such an intelligence which we have forgotten!

How often when we keep fit do we heed our internal organs? Yet without the "background operating system", or our involuntary Central Nervous System our organs would cease to function and we'd be dead!

We think as we suffer for example,

> "from heart failure or lie in a hospital bed, inactive with a pulse of over 160 beats a minute and poor circulation that it might help to start running? Do you think it would do the heart a favour by punishing it some more rather than teach it to relax and improve the way we breathe? "(Dr S. Chang)

Stress today is the major cause of illness and death. It affects the way we breathe as it becomes more shallow, consequently oxygenated blood is not being carried around the body as efficiently or carbon dioxide filtered efficiently from the blood either.

True To Our Roots: External Exercise Versus Internal Exercise!

According to Dr Chang, throughout its lifetime the heart is stimulated more by the "sympathetic nervous system, the voluntary nervous system, which originates in the spinal cord, than by the background operating system, or the involuntary nervous system, for example: anger, smoking, ball-games or horror films watching, stair-climbing and stimulating drinks, all accelerate the heart-rate - if exercise is added on to the burdens of the heart its chances of resting and gathering nutrients are greatly diminished."

True to our Roots or internal exercise is different as their main purpose is to relax the entire body so that the afflicted part can receive nourishment and heal itself.

Stress, anxiety, hypertension can be relieved by meridian stretching which we encourage through activating our fluid system, and enjoying deep and delicious fascial stretches, just like cats, dogs and other animals in nature.

Having been the strictest aerobic advocate for years I now finally begin to understand what the Chinese doctor told me when I was in my forties, at the height of my fitness career that my cardio-vascular system was depleting itself; that my heart and lungs needed a rest from all their over-activation. He was right, though at the time I didn't want to admit it as I used to run 400 meters in under two minutes daily, I developed asthma . . . I healed myself simply by practising gentle Qi Gong exercises and by stopping the running!!

It is as if we live in an era of the "fire" element. We need to exert ourselves, we have to sweat and get hot, otherwise we haven't done enough to . . . "look thinner, fitter, younger . . ."

The heart is connected to the fire element in Traditional Chinese Medicine - too much fire causes high blood

LESSON 6

pressure, heart attacks, congestion in the chest area, which also affects the lungs and the breath. This in turns affects the transportation of oxygenated blood to the rest of the body, when rigidity begins to set in. All because we have become stress junkies and thrive on excitable activities to feel alive.

An interesting note from a letter I received from The Finchley Clinic, London:

> *"Did you know?*
> *Exercise causes gut toxins to enter the blood and may make one feel lousy. Athletes who run for twenty minutes elevate their body temperature by 2 degrees Celsius. This increase in core heat increases gut permeability by 250%."*

While we are young it is evident that we are physically highly active and competitive, however this could be enhanced if children were reminded of good posture and how to use their feet when walking/running, therefore addressing the knee and hip alignment, which will also affect the pelvic and spinal health.

Posture is the basis of this ancient self-healing art, Qi Gong. When we hold ourselves well at all times, our fluid and energy system will flow undisturbed offering us better performance and avoiding possible future injuries.

Competitive sport is not something one should stop, but True to our Root's message is, incorporate the internal fluid work at the end of the sport, instead of forcing the cool-down stretches on already tight muscles. Recovery and flexibility will happen more efficiently while smoothing the accumulated lactic acid away.

True To Our Roots: External Exercise Versus Internal Exercise!

Introducing this method into cardio-vascular rehabilitation centres, and schools would be so precious! But then True to our Roots is a precious "tool" of which we only need a gentle reminder, as it is an inherited ability which we as the human race all possess.

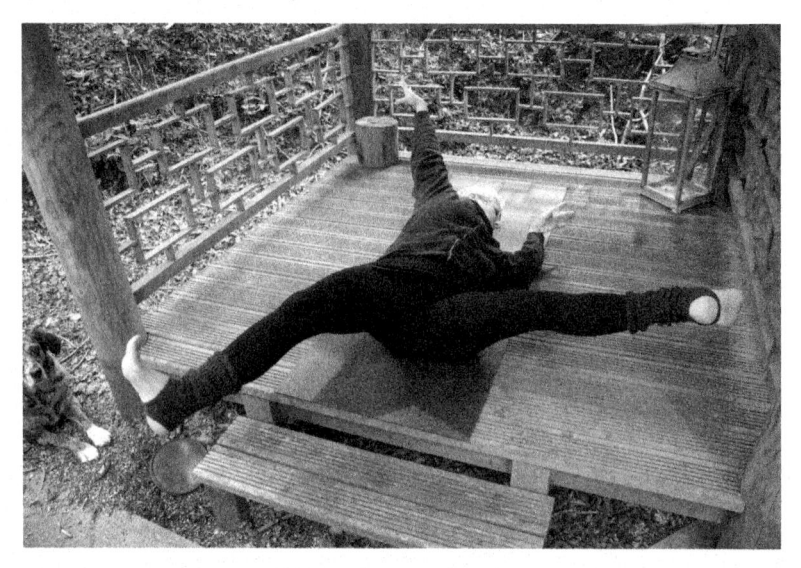

Practising Spontaneous Qi Gong, 2015

EPILOGUE.

EPILOGUE

How Did I Get These?

This little book may be focussing on us who suffer(ed) from osteo-arthritis, but I would like to think that the self-detective work can be applied for any other ailment, as this just represents the painting of each of our own individual lives.

Never ever give up on yourself, and always hope to create improvement in your self-belief.

After all, we are all in this together no matter what caste, creed or colour to eventually join forces when we depart from this material earth.

So, why not have fun with serenity and laugh ourselves through our sadnesses, knowing that "after the rains, the sun will shine again"!

BIBLIOGRAPHY.

Lesson 1.

- "Heal your Body", by Louise Hay
- Liz Koch: www.coreawareness.com Author of "The Psoas Book"
- Mr McMinn Surgeon and Inventor of the Hip Resurfacing procedure, Birmingham
- "Heal your Body", by Louise Hay

Lesson 2.

- "Heal your Body", by Louise Hay
- "Eight Steps to a Painfree Back", by Esther Gokhale
- Liz Koch: Application Course. www.coreawareness.com
- "Heal your Body", by Louise Hay

Lesson 3.

- "Out on a Limb", by Shirley MacLaine
- "Heal your Body", by Louise Hay

Lesson 4.

- "You can Heal your Life", by Louise Hay
- "The Revolutionary Trauma Release Process", by Dr David Berceli

- "Life on Land", by Emily Conrad (Founder of Continuum Movement: www.continuummovement.com)
- "Heal your Body", by Louise Hay

Lesson 5.

- "Leaving before the Rains Come", by Alexandra Fuller

Lesson 6.

- "The Complete System of Self-Healing Internal Exercises", by Dr Stephen Chang
- Quote taken from a letter received from The Finchley Clinic, London